THE ANTI-CANCER COOKBOOK

Healthy Recipes for Cancer Treatment and Recovery

Watson Lucas Felix

TABLE OF CONTENTS

Introduction

Conclusion

Copyright © 2023 Watson L. Felix

All rights reserved.

ISBN: 9798850506230

DEDICATION

This book is dedicated to God, my beloved family, whose unconditional love and support have been a source of infinite inspiration and strength. To my parents, my siblings, my husband, and my children—you are the reason for this book. Thank you for everything.

INTRODUCTION

The number one killer in the world is cancer. As a result, researchers and healthcare professionals have devoted a significant amount of time and effort to developing methods of treating and managing this deadly disease. One such method is dietary intervention. While specific diets or special food items may help fight cancer, the ultimate goal is to create a healthier nutrition plan tailored to the needs of individual cancer patients.

The Anti-Cancer Cookbook is a great resource for those looking to reduce their risk of cancer or dealing with cancer in the family. This cookbook provides delicious, easy-to-follow recipes designed for fighting five of the most common kinds of cancers - brain, breast, lung, prostate, and stomach. With these recipes, you can create personalized meal plans that take into account your dietary restrictions and lifestyle. Moreover, these recipes are packed with cancer-fighting ingredients and natural healing remedies, so you can make healthful, delicious meals that are both comforting and nourishing. So, let's get cooking and fight cancer with nutritious and tasty dishes!

This Cancer Diet Cookbook is filled with delicious, nutritious recipes specifically designed to give cancer fighters the nutrition they need while providing cancer-fighting benefits.

For the convenience of the reader, some of the recipes have been divided into sections based on the type of cancer with which they are associated. Each section gives tips on which foods are best for that particular type of cancer, as well as recipes that are tailored to the specific needs of cancer patients. In addition, readers will find ideas for meals and snacks, advice on dietary supplements, and other tips for making mealtime as enjoyable as possible.

The recipes in this cookbook are designed to help cancer fighters to make the right choices when it comes to their nutrition and to encourage them to eat delicious, nutritious food throughout their journey.

We wish you luck in your quest for a cancer-free life.

1.   RECIPES FOR BRAIN CANCER

When it comes to brain cancer, few medical treatment options are effective. This is why it is so important to focus on preventative measures that can help protect your brain health while still giving you delicious food options to choose from. A well-balanced diet with plenty of nutritious and wholesome food is essential to keeping your brain healthy. There are a few recipes that are specifically catered to brain cancer prevention and health. We will take a look at 5 of them in this article – Green Smoothie, Spinach Zucchini Lasagna, Curried Lentils, Cashew Poppy Seed Bites, and Quinoa Stuffed Squash.

Green Smoothie

The first recipe we will discuss is a green smoothie. This smoothie is an excellent source of several essential nutrients that every brain needs. It contains a blend of spinach, kale, celery, cucumber, avocado, and a banana. All of these ingredients are packed with antioxidants, vitamins, and minerals that help to protect your body from the damage of oxidative stress and free radicals. This smoothie is also rich in omega-3 fatty acids, which help to reduce inflammation and protect your brain from damage. To make the perfect green smoothie, start by blending the spinach and kale in a blender until smooth. Add in the remaining ingredients and blend until desired consistency is reached. Add a few drops of lemon juice and honey to give it a little natural sweetness. Enjoy this delicious smoothie every morning to protect your brain health.

Spinach Zucchini Lasagna

This delicious and hearty meal is packed with a variety of essential brain-boosting nutrients. Spinach is a good source of the antioxidant lutein, which helps protect your cells and reduce inflammation. Zucchini is a great source of magnesium, a mineral that helps to protect your neurons and promote neuroplasticity. To make this delicious lasagna, start by preheating the oven to 375F. In a pot, cook the spinach and zucchini until they are soft. Drain off any excess moisture. In a separate bowl, combine ricotta, Parmesan cheese, and eggs until well blended. To assemble the lasagna, layer the cooked spinach, zucchini, ricotta mixture, and tomato sauce. Sprinkle extra Parmesan cheese on top and bake in the preheated oven for 30 minutes or until the cheese is melted and golden brown. Enjoy this yummy dish that will protect your brain health with every bite.

Curried Lentils

Lentils are an excellent source of protein, which helps to reduce inflammation and protect your brain. This delicious and nutritious curried lentils recipe is full of flavor and spice. Start by sautéing onion, garlic, and ginger in a pan until the onion is soft. Add in the curry powder, cumin, and turmeric, and cook for a few minutes until fragrant. Then add in the lentils, vegetable broth, and diced tomatoes. Simmer for about 25 minutes until the lentils are cooked and the sauce has thickened. Finally, stir in some fresh cilantro for an extra burst of flavor. This delicious and nutritious dish will give your brain the protection it needs to stay healthy.

Cashew Poppy Seed Bites

These Cashew Poppy Seed Bites pack a punch of flavor and are easy to make. The cashews provide essential fatty acids, which help to reduce inflammation and protect your neurons. The poppy seeds are packed with magnesium, which helps to reduce oxidative stress and promote neuroplasticity. To make, start by adding the cashews, honey, and coconut oil to a food processor and blend until smooth. Form small balls of the mixture and roll in poppy seeds. Place in the refrigerator for one hour until set.

Enjoy these delicious, brain-protecting bites as a snack or a simple dessert.

Quinoa Stuffed Squash

Quinoa is an excellent source of protein, which helps to reduce inflammation and protect your neurons. This sweet and savory stuffed squash recipe is full of flavor and nutrition. Start by preheating the oven to 375F. Slice the squash in half and scoop out the seeds and discard. Place the squash halves onto a baking sheet and brush with olive oil. Bake for roughly 15 minutes in a preheated oven. While waiting, prepare the quinoa as directed on the package. In a separate pan, sauté onion and garlic in olive oil until soft. Add in mushrooms, spinach, chili pepper, and quinoa, and cook until vegetables are soft. Stuff the squash halves with the quinoa mixture and bake in the preheated oven for another 15 minutes. Enjoy this nutritious and delicious meal that will give your brain the protection it needs.

With all of these delicious and nutritious recipes, you and your brain will be getting the nutrition it needs to stay healthy and protected. All of these recipes are easy to make and medical research has proven that some of the ingredients used can reduce inflammation and improve brain health. When it comes to protecting your brain against cancer, it is never too late or too early to start taking steps to improve your brain health. Eating these brain-healthy meals can help you do just that and give you delicious food options you can enjoy guilt-free.

2.   RECIPES FOR BREAST CANCER

With the number of cases of breast cancer on the rise, it's important to introduce better-eating habits into one's lifestyle. Eating nutritious meals can help reduce the risk of developing breast cancer, and for patients already facing the disease, it's imperative to take into consideration nutrition to help support the body during treatment. Eating a balanced diet with meals including foods rich in vitamins, minerals, and anti-inflammatory properties is key to ensuring that the body has the necessary nutrients it needs. That is why we have put together five delicious and healthy recipes that are ideal for individuals fighting breast cancer.

Avocado Egg Salad

Avocado Egg Salad is one of the most popular recipes for encouraging breast cancer prevention. It is rich in healthy fats and proteins which help to reduce the risk of breast cancer. To create this recipe, you'll need the following ingredients: four hard-boiled eggs, two avocados, one lemon, one tablespoon of olive oil, salt, and pepper.

First, remove the eggshells from the hard-boiled eggs. Cut the eggs into small cubes and mix them with two avocados that have been diced and mashed into a smooth paste. Squeeze the lemon juice into the mixture and add olive oil, salt, and pepper to taste. Serve this salad cold or warm.

Kale and Quinoa Salad

Kale and quinoa are two highly nutritious ingredients that are delicious when combined. Not only is this a tasty dish, but it is also a great option for those fighting breast cancer. Kale is rich in antioxidants which help to reduce inflammation. Quinoa is also high in protein and helps to provide the body with essential minerals and vitamins. To make this salad, you'll need the following ingredients: one cup of quinoa, two cups of chopped kale, two tablespoons of olive oil, lemon juice, salt, and pepper.

Start by rinsing the quinoa using a strainer and then bring it to a boil over medium heat. Let the quinoa simmer, stirring occasionally for about fifteen minutes. Once cooked, remove the quinoa from the heat and set aside to cool.

In a large bowl, combine two cups of chopped kale and the cooled quinoa. Drizzle the mixture with two tablespoons of olive oil and stir. Let the salad cool before adding a squeeze of lemon juice, salt, and pepper to taste. Serve this salad chilled or at room temperature.

Roasted Mediterranean Vegetables

This delicious roasted vegetable dish is perfect for those looking for a healthy meal to reduce their risk of breast cancer. It contains a variety of vegetables that are rich in antioxidants, vitamins, and minerals. The vegetables in this dish are also known to reduce inflammation and help to strengthen the immune system. This recipe includes ingredients such as one zucchini, one red bell pepper, one eggplant, two tablespoons of olive oil, and one tablespoon of rosemary, salt, and pepper.

Start by setting your oven to 375°F before preparing this dish. While the oven is preheating, chop the zucchini, red bell pepper, and eggplant into small cubes. Spread the vegetables over a baking sheet, and top with two tablespoons of olive oil and one tablespoon of rosemary. Sprinkle salt and pepper to taste. Bake the vegetables for thirty minutes, flipping them over halfway through the cooking process. Once cooked, remove from the oven and enjoy as a side dish or on its own.

Coconut Chicken Curry

Coconut Chicken Curry is a tasty Indian dish that is packed with health benefits. This meal is rich in proteins and spices that help to boost the immune system and reduce inflammation. Coconut milk is high in antioxidants and helps to provide much-needed vitamins and minerals to the body. This Coconut Chicken Curry recipe consists of the following ingredients: four chicken breasts, one cup of coconut milk, one teaspoon of turmeric, one teaspoon of garam masala, two tablespoons of olive oil, and salt to taste.

Begin by marinating the chicken with a teaspoon of each turmeric and garam masala for twenty minutes. Heat two tablespoons of olive oil in a saucepan over medium-high heat. Once heated, add the marinated chicken to the pan and cook for ten minutes, stirring occasionally. Next, add one cup of coconut milk and bring to a simmer. Reduce the heat and simmer for an additional twenty minutes. Once the chicken is cooked through, remove the curry from the heat and serve with rice or bread.

Turkey Burgers

Turkey Burgers are a great option for anyone looking to reduce their risk of breast cancer. Turkey is low in fat but high in proteins and vitamins, making it a perfect meal for those fighting cancer. To create your turkey burgers, you'll need the following ingredients: one pound of ground turkey, one teaspoon of rosemary, one teaspoon of garlic powder, one egg, and salt and pepper.

Preheat your oven to 350°F. In a large bowl, mix one pound of ground turkey, one teaspoon of rosemary, one teaspoon of garlic powder, one egg, and salt and pepper to taste. Form the turkey mixture into four burger patties. Place the patties on a cooking sheet and bake in the oven for twenty minutes. Serve these burgers with lettuce, tomato, onion, and your favorite condiments.

These five delicious recipes for people fighting breast cancer are sure to be a hit in any home kitchen. By incorporating these recipes into your meal plan, you can ensure that you're getting all the nutrition you need to fight breast cancer. By making healthier eating choices, you can help to reduce the risk of developing breast cancer.

3. RECIPES FOR LUNG CANCER

Lung cancer is the leading cause of cancer-related death in the world, and recent statistics reveal that the mortality rate is expected to rise even further. fighting off cancer can be a real challenge, as lung cancer treatments often produce uncomfortable and even painful side effects. Treatment isn't the only way to help your body heal. Eating the right foods is also essential to maintain your health.

Here are some recipes that are packed with a nutritious punch, while also tasting great. They are designed to help build your immune system, fight inflammation, and even reduce symptoms related to lung cancer.

Fish Tacos with Mango Slaw

This tropical-inspired fish tacos dish makes for a light yet filling lunch or dinner. Not only does the tropical mango slaw bring a unique flavor and texture to the tacos, but it's also full of nutrients. The mango contains powerful antioxidants such as vitamins A, C, and E, which can help reduce inflammation in the body. The anti-inflammatory powers combined with the omega-3 fatty acids in the fish make this dish a great option for those with lung cancer.

Ingredients:

• 2 cups cooked white fish

• 1 mango, chopped

• 3/4 cup chopped red onion

• 2 tablespoons diced jalapeño (optional)

• 1/4 cup chopped fresh cilantro

• 2 tablespoons olive oil

• Juice of 1 lime

• Salt and pepper, to taste

• 6 corn tortillas

Instructions:

1. In a medium-sized bowl, mix the mango, red onion, jalapeno (if using), and cilantro.

2. Drizzle with the olive oil and lime juice and season with salt and pepper, stirring to combine.

3. Heat a skillet over medium heat and add the cooked fish. Heat until warmed through.

4. Using a slotted spoon, remove the fish from a plate.

5. Add the tortillas to the warm skillet and heat, flipping once, until lightly browned.

6. To assemble, divide the fish, mango slaw, and optional toppings among the tortillas. Enjoy!

Roasted Garlic Soup

This hearty and flavorful soup is a great comfort meal for those with lung cancer. Roasted garlic provides plenty of antioxidants, as well as anti-inflammatory, anti-cancer, and immune-boosting properties. The lentils provide an extra boost of plant protein and fiber for sustained energy throughout the day.

Ingredients:

- 1 head of garlic

- 2 tablespoons olive oil

- 1 medium onion, chopped

- 2 carrots, peeled and chopped

- 2 stalks of celery, chopped

- 1 teaspoon dried oregano

- 1 teaspoon dried thyme

- 1 lentil, rinsed

- 4 cups vegetable broth

- Salt and pepper, to taste

Instructions:

1. Preheat oven to 400°F (200°C).

2. Peel away the outer layers of the garlic head, leaving the cloves intact.

3. Cut the top of the garlic head off and place the head cut-side up onto a piece of aluminum foil. Drizzle olive oil over the top and wrap the head in the foil.

4. Roast the garlic in the preheated oven for 25 minutes.

5. Heat another 2 tablespoons olive oil in a large pot over medium heat.

6. Add the onion, carrots, and celery and cook for 7 minutes until vegetables have softened.

7. Add the oregano and thyme and stir until combined.

8. Squeeze the roasted garlic cloves out of the head of garlic into the pot and stir.

9. Add the lentil and vegetable broth and bring the soup to a boil.

10. Simmer for 30 minutes at reduced heat.

11. Remove from heat and let cool.

12. Blend the soup with an immersion blender until it's smooth.

13. Add salt and pepper to taste. Enjoy!

Roasted Cauliflower Soup

Cauliflower is a cruciferous vegetable, meaning it has high levels of cancer-fighting antioxidants. This roasted cauliflower soup is full of flavor and a great way to incorporate more cruciferous vegetables into your diet. The lemon provides a bright citrus flavor and an extra boost of Vitamin C to the soup, which helps reduce inflammation.

Ingredients:

• 1 cauliflower head, cut into florets

• 2 tablespoons olive oil

• 2 cloves garlic, minced

• 1 small onion, chopped

- 1 teaspoon dried thyme

- 3 cups vegetable broth

- Juice of 1 lemon

- Salt and pepper, to taste

Instructions:

1. Preheat oven to 400°F (200°C).

2. Spread the chopped cauliflower florets on a baking sheet.

3. Olive oil should be added along with salt and pepper.

4. Roast in the preheated oven for 30 minutes, stirring once halfway through.

5. Heat the remaining 2 tablespoons of olive oil in a large pot over medium heat.

6. Add the garlic, onion, and thyme, and cook for 5 minutes until the vegetables have softened.

7. Add the roasted cauliflower and vegetable broth to the pot and bring to a boil.

8. Simmer for 15 minutes on low heat.

9. Add the lemon juice and stir to combine.

10. Using an immersion blender, blend the soup until smooth.

11. Add salt and pepper to taste. Enjoy!

Quinoa and Kale Bowl

This flavorful and healthy quinoa bowl is like a burst of sunshine in your mouth. The combination of grains, legumes, and veggies makes it a complete dish for those with lung cancer. Quinoa and kale are both nutritional powerhouses, providing ample amounts of protein, fiber, vitamins, and minerals.

Ingredients:

- 1 cup cooked quinoa

- 2 cups kale, chopped

- 1/2 cup cooked black beans

- 1/2 cup cherry tomatoes, halved

- 2 tablespoons diced red onions

- 2 tablespoons olive oil

- Juice of 1/2 lemon

- Salt and pepper, to taste

Instructions:

1. In a medium-sized bowl, combine the quinoa, kale, black beans, tomatoes, and onions.

2. Drizzle with the olive oil and lemon juice and toss until everything is evenly coated.

3. Season with salt and pepper and mix once more.

4. Serve in a bowl and enjoy!

Zucchini Noodles with Pesto

This veggie-packed dish is simple but packs a lot of flavor. The spiralized zucchini noodles provide a light alternative to heavier pasta noodles, and they offer a great source of vitamins and minerals. The pesto is full of healthy fats from olive oil and pine nuts, which can help reduce inflammation and protect the body against cancer cells.

Ingredients:

• 4 zucchini, spiralized

• 2 cloves garlic, minced

• 2 tablespoons pine nuts

• 2 tablespoons freshly grated Parmesan cheese

• 3 tablespoons olive oil

• Juice of 1/2 lemon

• Salt and pepper, to taste

Instructions:

1. Heat a large skillet over medium heat and add the garlic and pine nuts. About 1-2 minutes of stirring is needed until the mixture is lightly roasted.

2. Add the spiralized zucchini noodles and cook for 5 minutes, stirring occasionally, until the noodles are lightly cooked.

3. Take out of the heat and place on a plate.

4. In a food processor or blender, blend the Parmesan cheese, olive oil, and lemon juice until a thick pesto forms.

5. Toss the cooked noodles with the pesto and season with salt and pepper. Enjoy!

All of these recipes are designed to provide you with the optimum nutrition you need to fight lung cancer. While everyone is different, it's important to find a dietary plan that works for you. Incorporating these dishes into your meals can help you feel better and stronger every day.

4. RECIPES FOR PROSTATE CANCER

Prostate cancer is one of the most common cancers among men and for good reason. Many lifestyle factors make it more likely for men to be diagnosed with the disease. To reduce the risk of developing prostate cancer, men should make an effort to maintain a healthy diet. Foods high in omega-3s, such as fatty fish, and those with antioxidants, such as dark green vegetables, are recommended choices. For men already undergoing treatment for prostate cancer, a diet rich in vitamins and minerals, low in saturated fats and unrefined carbohydrates, and rich in protein is essential. Below are five delicious recipes specifically tailored to meet a prostate cancer diet.

Roasted Butternut Squash with Lentils

This hearty dish is packed with protein from both lentils and squash, as well as plenty of antioxidants and fiber. It's a simple dish to prepare and can be enjoyed as a hearty main course or side dish.

Ingredients:

-1 medium butternut squash

-1 onion

-1 cup of dry lentils

-1 tablespoon of olive oil

-1 teaspoon of salt and pepper

-1 tablespoon of ground cumin

-½ teaspoon of ground ginger

-2 tablespoons of balsamic vinegar

Instructions:

1. Preheat the oven to 400°F.

2. Peel and deseed the butternut squash, then cut into ½-inch cubes.

3. Thinly slice the onion.

4. In a medium pot, bring 2 cups of water to a boil and add the lentils. Cook the lentils for 15-20 minutes until they are tender.

5. In a large baking dish, combine the cubed squash, sliced onion, and cooked lentils.

6. Drizzle with olive oil and season with salt, pepper, cumin, and ginger.

7. Bake in the preheated oven for 25-30 minutes, stirring halfway through, until the squash is tender.

8. Drizzle the roasted vegetables with balsamic vinegar and serve.

Greek Quinoa Bowl

This tasty bowl is packed with Greek-inspired flavors and healthy ingredients like quinoa, diced tomatoes, cucumber, and feta cheese. It's a great source of protein and fiber and can make a healthy, filling lunch or light dinner.

Ingredients:

-1 cup of uncooked quinoa

-2 cups of vegetable broth

-1 large tomato, diced

-1 large cucumber, diced

-¼ cup of crumbled feta cheese

-¼ cup of pitted olives

-1 tablespoon of olive oil

-2 tablespoons of freshly squeezed lemon juice

-1 tablespoon of dried oregano

-Salt and pepper to taste

Instructions:

1. In a medium pot, bring the vegetable broth to a boil and add the quinoa. Quinoa will become tender after 15 minutes of simmering on low heat.

2. Meanwhile, in a large bowl, combine the diced tomatoes, cucumber, feta cheese, and olives. Drizzle the mixture with the olive oil, lemon juice, oregano, and salt and pepper.

3. Once the quinoa is cooked, add it to the bowl of vegetables and mix to combine.

4. Serve the Greek quinoa bowl warm or chilled.

Veggie-Loaded Quesadillas

These flavorful vegetarian quesadillas are packed with healthy ingredients like spinach, bell peppers, onions, and jalapeños. The combination of cheese and vegetables make them a filling and tasty dish.

Ingredients:

-6 whole wheat or corn tortillas

-1 onion, finely chopped

-1 bell pepper, chopped

-1 jalapeño, chopped

-2 cups of spinach

-2 cups of shredded cheese

-1 tablespoon of olive oil

-Salt and pepper to taste

Instructions:

1. A big skillet with medium heat is used to warm the olive oil.

2. Add the onion, bell pepper, and jalapeño to the pan and cook until the vegetables are tender about 5 minutes.

3. Add the spinach to the skillet and season with salt and pepper. Cook for 2 minutes, or until the spinach is wilted.

4. Spread the vegetable mixture on one-half of each of the tortillas.

5. Top with the shredded cheese and fold the empty half of each tortilla over the top.

6. Cook the quesadillas on a large skillet over medium heat until the cheese is melted and the tortillas are golden, about 3-5 minutes per side.

7. Cut each quesadilla into 4 slices and serve.

Lentil and Avocado Salad

This protein-packed salad offers a great combination of flavors and textures. It's a great lunch or side dish to accompany any meal.

Ingredients:

-1 cup of uncooked lentils

-2 cups of water

-1 avocado, diced

-1 cup of cherry tomatoes, halved

-1 cucumber, diced

-¼ cup of chopped cilantro

-2 tablespoons of freshly squeezed lime juice

-1 tablespoon of olive oil

-Salt and pepper to taste

Instructions:

1. In a medium pot, bring 2 cups of water to a boil and add the lentils. Till the lentils are cooked, simmer for 15 to 20 minutes.

2. In a large bowl, combine the cooked lentils, diced avocado, cherry tomatoes, cucumber, and cilantro.

3. Drizzle with the lime juice and olive oil, and season with salt and pepper.

4. Toss to combine and serve.

Grilled Salmon with Sautéed Veggies

This delicious and healthy dish is packed with vitamins, minerals, and omega-3 fatty acids, which are beneficial for prostate health. It's a perfect dinner for any night of the week.

Ingredients:

-2 salmon fillets

-1 tablespoon of olive oil

-Salt and pepper to taste

-1 onion, chopped

-1 red bell pepper, chopped

-1 yellow bell pepper, chopped

-1 zucchini, chopped

-2 tablespoons of balsamic vinegar

Instructions:

1. A big skillet with medium heat is used to warm the olive oil.

2. Season the salmon fillets with salt and pepper, and place in the skillet. Cook for 3–4 minutes on each side or until thoroughly done.

3. The salmon should be taken out of the pan and placed aside.

4. In the same pan, add the onion, bell peppers, and zucchini. Vegetables should be sautéed for 5-7 minutes, or until they are soft and slightly browned.

5. Drizzle the vegetables with the balsamic vinegar and season with salt and pepper.

6. Serve the salmon alongside the sautéed vegetables.

These five recipes are a great way to meet the dietary needs of those with prostate cancer. With delicious, healthy ingredients and easy-to-follow instructions, they make it easy for anyone to get the necessary nutrients needed to aid in the treatment of prostate cancer.

5. RECIPES FOR STOMACH CANCER

Stomach cancer is one of the deadliest forms of cancer and unfortunately, there is no known cure. However, maintaining a healthy lifestyle and eating nutritious meals can help reduce the risk of developing this dreadful disease. A balanced diet is key when it comes to cancer prevention and one of the best ways to ensure this is to incorporate delicious and nourishing recipes into your daily meals. In this article, we will provide five recipes for stomach cancer that are not only nutritious and delicious, but also easy to make. Each of these recipes is packed with nutrients that will help fight stomach cancer and support overall health. Read on for five recipes that are sure to please and nourish your body.

Recipe 1: Creamy Butternut Squash Soup

This creamy butternut squash soup is high in fiber and antioxidants; both of which can help reduce the risk of developing stomach cancer. The squash is cooked until tender and blended along with deliciously creamy ingredients like Greek yogurt, nutmeg, and garlic to create an unbelievably flavorful and nourishing soup.

Ingredients:

-1 butternut squash, peeled, seeded, and diced

-1 tablespoon olive oil

-1 onion, finely diced

-2 cloves of garlic, minced

-2 cups vegetable broth

-1/2 teaspoon ground nutmeg

-1/2 teaspoon ground cinnamon

-1/4 cup Greek yogurt

-Salt and pepper, to taste

Instructions:

1. In a big pot set over medium heat, warm the oil.

2. Add the onion and garlic and cook until soft and fragrant, about 5 minutes.

3. Add the butternut squash and cook until softened, about 5 minutes more.

4. Pour in the vegetable broth and add the nutmeg and cinnamon. Bring to a boil and then reduce the heat and simmer until the squash is tender, about 10 minutes.

5. Working in batches, transfer the soup to a blender and blend until creamy. Return the soup to the pot and add the Greek yogurt and season with salt and pepper, to taste.

6. Serve warm.

Recipe 2: Mediterranean Quinoa Salad

This fantastic Mediterranean quinoa salad is not only full of nutritious ingredients but also incredibly flavorful. It contains heart-healthy olive oil, antioxidant-rich tomatoes, and protein-packed quinoa, making it an excellent choice for those at risk of developing stomach cancer.

Ingredients:

-1 cup quinoa

-2 cups vegetable broth

-1 cup cherry tomatoes, halved

-1/2 cup Kalamata olives, pitted and chopped

-1/2 cup feta cheese, crumbled

-1/4 cup freshly chopped parsley

-1/4 cup olive oil

-1/4 cup freshly squeezed lemon juice

-1 clove of garlic, minced

-Salt and pepper, to taste

Instructions:

1. In a medium saucepan, combine the quinoa and vegetable broth and bring to a boil. Reduce the heat and simmer until the quinoa is cooked through about 15 minutes.

2. In a large bowl, combine the cooked quinoa, tomatoes, olives, feta cheese, and parsley.

3. In a separate bowl, whisk together the olive oil, lemon juice, garlic, salt, and pepper.

4. After adding the dressing, incorporate the quinoa mixture by tossing.

5. Serve chilled or at room temperature.

Recipe 3: Roasted Cauliflower Steaks

These tasty roasted cauliflower steaks are easy to make and packed with nutrients that can help reduce the risk of stomach cancer. The cauliflower is seasoned with herbs and garlic to provide a delicious flavor and then roasted to perfection for a deliciously healthy side dish.

Ingredients:

- 1 head of cauliflower, cut into 4 steaks

- 1 tablespoon olive oil

- 1 teaspoon dried oregano

- 1 teaspoon garlic powder

- Salt and pepper, to taste

Instructions:

1. Set the oven's temperature to 400 degrees.

2. Place the cauliflower steaks in a single layer on a baking pan and drizzle with olive oil.

3. Sprinkle the oregano, garlic powder, salt, and pepper over the cauliflower.

4. Roast in the preheated oven for 20 minutes or until golden and tender.

5. Serve hot.

Recipe 4: Baked Salmon with Salsa

This delectable baked salmon is full of lean protein and healthy fats that can help prevent stomach cancer. The salmon is marinated to perfection and topped with fresh salsa for a burst of flavor in every bite.

Ingredients:

- Cut a one-pound salmon fillet into four halves.

-3 tablespoons olive oil

-3 cloves of garlic, minced

-2 tablespoons freshly squeezed lemon juice

-1 teaspoon dried oregano

-Salt and pepper, to taste

-For the salsa:

-1 cup cherry tomatoes, chopped

-1/2 cup finely chopped red onion

-1/4 cup freshly chopped cilantro

-1 tablespoon freshly squeezed lime juice

-Salt and pepper, to taste

Instructions:

1. 375 degrees Fahrenheit should be the oven's temperature setting.

2. Place the salmon in a baking dish and pour the olive oil over it. Sprinkle the garlic, lemon juice, oregano, salt, and pepper over the salmon.

3. Bake in the preheated oven for 15 minutes or until the salmon is cooked through.

4. Meanwhile, prepare the salsa by combining the cherry tomatoes, red onion, cilantro, lime juice, salt, and pepper in a medium bowl.

5. Once the salmon Is cooked, top each portion with the salsa and serve.

Recipe 5: Apple Crumble

This scrumptious apple crumble is a tasty and nutritious dessert that is so easy to make. It is packed with fiber-rich apples, oats, and almonds, creating a deliciously healthy snack or dessert.

Ingredients:

-4 apples, peeled, cored, and diced

-1/4 cup light brown sugar

-1 teaspoon ground cinnamon

-2 tablespoons butter

-1/2 cup quick-cooking oats

-1/2 cup almond meal

-1/4 teaspoon ground nutmeg

-1/4 cup maple syrup

Instructions:

1. 350 degrees Fahrenheit should be the oven's temperature setting.

2. Place the apples in an 8-inch baking dish and sprinkle with the brown sugar and cinnamon.

3. Dot the apples with the butter.

4. In a medium bowl, combine the oats, almond meal, nutmeg, and maple syrup. Sprinkle the mixture over the apples.

5. Bake in the preheated oven for 40 minutes or until the crumble is golden and the apples are tender.

6. Serve warm.

Conclusion

Stomach cancer is a serious form of cancer that requires both prevention and knowledge to reduce the risk. Eating

a healthy and balanced diet is key to reducing the risk and incorporating recipes such as these five options can provide your body with the nutrition it needs to fight off the disease. From creamy butternut squash soup to apple crumble, these delicious recipes are sure to please and provide you with the nourishment necessary to help prevent stomach cancer.

6.   DIETARY SUPPLEMENT TIPS

Cancer is a complicated condition that can be challenging to manage. For many cancer patients, complementary treatment options such as dietary supplements are an important part of their comprehensive cancer care plan. Dietary supplements, which are vitamins, minerals, herbs, and other substances taken in pill or capsule form, can help your body manage the side effects of treatments and promote overall health and a sense of well-being. It is important to know, however, that dietary supplements should be used in moderation and should never be used as a substitute for conventional medical treatments like chemotherapy or radiation. There are some key things to keep in mind when considering dietary supplements for cancer.

Dietary supplements may be beneficial for cancer patients because they can:

• Boost the immune system

• Improve digestion, absorption, and assimilation of nutrients

• Reduce inflammation

• Reduce side effects from cancer treatments, such as nausea, fatigue, and radiation dermatitis

What Types of Supplements Can Help?

When it comes to cancer, certain dietary supplements may provide some benefits. Vitamins, minerals, and certain herbs have all been studied for their potential benefits in cancer patients.

Vitamins

Vitamins are essential for many of your body's functions, and taking vitamins can help support your health during cancer treatments. Commonly-taken vitamins include vitamin A, to help support cells, and C and E, which are antioxidants that neutralize free radicals to help keep cells healthy. Folic acid is also thought to be beneficial, as it helps with DNA replication, which can in turn help with cell growth.

Minerals

Minerals are also essential for various body functions and include iron, magnesium, and selenium. Iron helps create red blood cells and can help counter fatigue; magnesium helps support healthy cell structure, and selenium is another antioxidant that helps protect cells.

Herbs

Herbs have a wide array of potential benefits for cancer patients. Many herbs possess antioxidants that can help protect cells, while others may help boost the immune system. According to the American Cancer Society, some herbs may even be able to kill cancer cells directly. Common herbs for cancer include turmeric, green tea extract, and ashwagandha.

Other Dietary Supplements

Some other dietary supplements can also be beneficial for those with cancer. Omega-3 fatty acids, for example, are thought to be able to reduce inflammation and enhance immune system response. Coenzyme Q10 is another substance that has some antioxidant activity and may also be symbiotic with chemotherapy treatments.

How Do I Take Dietary Supplements?

When taking dietary supplements, it is important to remember that they should be used in moderation. Too much of any vitamin, mineral, or herb can cause problems, so be sure to use them only as directed. Additionally, it is important to remember that dietary

supplements are not a substitute for conventional cancer treatments. Dietary supplements may provide some benefits, but they should always be used in conjunction with conventional treatments.

It is also important to discuss any dietary supplements with your doctor. Different types of dietary supplements may interact with each other or with other medications you are taking, such as those for chemotherapy or radiation. Your doctor can help you identify potential interactions and adjust your dosage appropriately.

Tips for Selecting Dietary Supplements

When selecting dietary supplements, it is important to make sure you are getting high-quality products. Some tips to help ensure that you are getting the best possible ingredients are:

- Check for third-party certification – Supplements with certification, such as the U.S. Pharmacopoeia or Good Manufacturing Practices seal, indicating that the product has been tested and meets certain standards for potency and purity.

- Buy from reputable sources – Make sure to purchase your supplements from a reputable retailer or manufacturer.

- Don't mix and match – Avoid buying different brands of the same type of supplement, as they may contain different doses or ingredients.

Dietary supplements can be a great complement to traditional cancer treatments. However, it is important to research different types of supplements and discuss them with your doctor. Be sure to look for high-quality options and use them in moderation, and never use dietary supplements as a substitute for conventional cancer treatment.

Other dietary supplement tips for cancer patients.

Finding the Right Supplement

The first tip for cancer patients is to find the right supplement. As mentioned above, there are a variety of dietary supplements that can be beneficial for cancer patients. Some of the most popular supplements include turmeric, ginger, probiotics, omega-3 fatty acids, and vitamin D. It is important to talk to your healthcare professional before taking any supplement to make sure that it will not interact with any medications or treatments. Your healthcare team can also help you identify the right type of supplement based on your specific needs.

Take High-Quality Supplements

The second tip for cancer patients is to take only high-quality supplements. Dietary supplements are not subject to the same regulations as medications, so it is important to make sure that you are taking only safe and effective products. Look for supplements that have been tested and certified by a third-party organization, such as the US Pharmacopeia (USP) or Consumer Labs, which are two of the most reputable organizations. All certified supplements should contain the USP seal of approval on the label.

Follow the Recommended Dosage

The third tip for cancer patients is to follow the recommended dosage. It is important to take dietary supplements as directed by your healthcare provider. Each type of supplement may have different dosage instructions, so it is important to follow these instructions carefully. Overdosing supplements can have dangerous consequences, so it is important to talk to your doctor before increasing the dose.

Talk to Your Doctors

The fourth tip for cancer patients is to talk to your healthcare team. Many supplements can interfere with the effectiveness of traditional cancer treatments, such as chemotherapy and radiation. Therefore, it is important to talk to your doctor before taking any type of supplement. Your healthcare team can help you find the right balance between supplements and treatments to get the most benefit.

Supplementation and Prevention

The fifth and final tip for cancer patients is to supplement for prevention. Dietary supplements can be an effective tool for prevention and early detection of cancer. There is some evidence that suggests certain supplements can help reduce the risk of developing certain types of cancer, such as colorectal, bladder, and prostate cancer. However, due to the lack of clinical trials, there is no definitive answer about the effectiveness of supplements for cancer prevention. Therefore, it is important to talk to your healthcare team before taking any supplement for prevention.

Dietary supplements can be an important part of cancer care. Supplements can help boost the immune system, improve digestion and absorption of nutrients, reduce inflammation, and reduce side effects related to cancer treatments. However, it is important to find the right supplement and use it properly. Talk to your doctor before taking any supplement and always make sure to take only high-quality products. Following these dietary supplement tips can help cancer patients get the most benefit from their supplements.

CONCLUSION

The Anti-Cancer Cookbook has provided an invaluable resource in presenting recipes for brain, breast, lung, prostate, and stomach cancers, as well as dietary supplement tips. All of these recipes offer important nutrients and anti-cancer power foods, which can help combat cancer symptoms and boost the body's healing potential. Additionally, the dietary supplement tips offer further options for those looking for additional support in their fight against cancer. We hope this book has been useful in helping you find the right recipes for each type of cancer and the right dietary supplement tips to ensure that you have the best possible chance of fighting cancer.

ABOUT THE AUTHOR

I specialize in self-help, health, and fitness writing. I have been passionate about health and wellness for all of my life and helping others pursue healthier, happier, and more satisfying lives is what motivates me daily. I love to dive into health and fitness topics to help readers connect with the material in a more personal way. As a long-time personal trainer, group fitness instructor, and healthy lifestyle advocate I feel that I have the knowledge and experience to share tips, stories, and insights. As an inspiring motivator, I empower my readers and help them live an active, fulfilling life.

www.ingramcontent.com/pod-product-compliance
Lightning Source LLC
Chambersburg PA
CBHW070215260726
48658CB00006BA/2086